Depression, are you OK?

Can you win the battle against anxiety and depression?

Dr. Lucy Coleman

COLEMAN PUBLISHING

Coleman Publishing

For permission requests, please contact:

Email: info@lifebosshealth.com

10 9 8 7 6 5 4 3 2 1

ISBN: 978-1-949545-12-8

Contents

Introduction

The fog

Depression. Anxiety. Fear.

These words echo through the lives of millions of people every single day. They are more than just clinical terms—they are lived realities. Silent weights carried in minds and hearts around the world. Depression has become one of the leading causes of suicide, relationship breakdowns, chronic illness, and a diminishing quality of life across every age group and culture.

Today, more people than ever have access to information about mental health—yet many still feel lost. The internet overflows with articles and videos that often highlight the problem more than the solution. If you've found yourself overwhelmed by what you've read or heard, if you feel discouraged or hopeless, please know this: *you are not alone, and there is a path forward*.

This book is not just about naming the pain. It is about breaking free from it.

Depression is not always caused by a single event or easily identifiable factor. In reality, it often arises from a complex web of emotional, psychological, environmental, biological, and even chemical influences. For some, it is rooted in unresolved trauma—such as childhood neglect, abuse, or the impact of a deeply painful experience that continues to echo through their life. For others, depression may begin after a significant loss: the death of a loved one, the end of a meaningful relationship, the loss of a job, or a sudden shift in identity or purpose.

Long-term stress, burnout, or constant exposure to toxic environments—whether at work, in family dynamics, or within social circles—can wear down emotional resilience. Loneliness, isolation, and a lack of supportive connection also commonly contribute to the onset of depressive symptoms.

Biological factors, such as hormonal imbalances (postpartum, perimenopause, thyroid dysfunction), chronic illnesses, or neurological conditions, can create fertile ground for depression to take hold. In some cases, even medications—especially those affecting brain chemistry, such as certain birth control pills, blood pressure medications, sleep aids, corticosteroids, or medications for chronic pain—can induce or worsen depressive episodes as a side effect.

Genetics also play a role; individuals with a family history of depression may carry a greater vulnerability, even if their external circumstances appear stable. Meanwhile, poor nutrition, substance abuse, and lack of restorative sleep can silently deplete the body and mind, lowering resistance to emotional challenges.

Depression can also emerge quietly, without an obvious cause—sometimes a slow, creeping fog that builds until it becomes difficult to recognize yourself. This is what makes depression so misunderstood, and why compassion and awareness are so essential in addressing it.

Understanding these diverse causes is not about placing blame; it's about recognizing that depression is real, multifaceted, and valid—regardless of its origin. And knowing this opens the door to healing, because true healing must be just as personal, layered, and compassionate as the path that led there.

In the chapters ahead, you'll gain more than just an understanding of what depression and anxiety are. You'll learn how they affect your body, your emotions, and your relationships—and most importantly, what you can do about them. This book offers practical tools, empowering perspectives, and long-term strategies to move you toward a place of emotional resilience, calm, and fulfillment.

Think of this book as your roadmap to inner freedom. Whether you're struggling with depression, recovering from anxiety, or simply feeling emotionally drained, these pages were written for *you*. Here, you will find guidance, not judgment. Encouragement, not pressure. Compassion, not cliché.

No matter how dark things may feel right now, know that better days are possible. You are not broken. You are human—and healing is within reach.

So let this be a new beginning. Approach each chapter with an open heart and a willingness to learn. Allow yourself to reflect, to feel, and to change. Yes, you may have endured difficult moments in the past—but your story is far from over. There are still dreams to live, relationships to nourish, peace to rediscover, and joy to reclaim.

When you reach the final chapter, you won't just be more informed—you'll be more equipped. You'll carry with you the tools, mindsets, and practices that empower you to reclaim your life and shape a brighter, more balanced future.

Are you ready to begin?

Take a deep breath. Lift your chin. Offer yourself kindness. And take the first step into a space where healing begins and hope becomes real.

Chapter 1

Understanding depression and anxiety - two sides of the same coin

Imagine this: something shocking or heartbreaking happens in your life. A job loss. A betrayal. A frightening diagnosis. In the hours or days that follow, you feel shaken, sad, or scared. These emotional reactions are natural responses to difficult events. But when these feelings persist, intensify, or begin to take over your daily life, they may point to something more serious—depression or anxiety.

Many people think of depression as simply "feeling sad," and anxiety as "worrying too much." But these conditions are far more complex. Depression can present as a quiet erosion of joy, energy, and motivation. Anxiety can manifest as relentless worry, inner tension, or panic—sometimes with no clear cause. And often, they walk hand in hand. Depression can trigger anxiety, and chronic anxiety can spiral into depression. This overlap is why they're often treated together.

What exactly is depression?

Depression is a mental health disorder that affects the way you feel, think, act, and function. It is more than temporary sadness—it's a persistent cloud that interferes with your ability to enjoy life, make decisions, and carry out daily responsibilities.

Depression is frequently misunderstood as a weakness or a character flaw. It's not. It is a real and treatable condition often rooted in neurochemical imbalances, unresolved trauma, or accumulated stress. Depression can be triggered by:

- A significant loss or trauma

- Chronic stress or burnout

- Physical illness or chronic pain

- Social isolation or loneliness

- Genetics or family history

- Substance abuse

- Postpartum hormonal shifts

- Life transitions (divorce, relocation, retirement)

- Even certain medications—such as corticosteroids, hormonal treatments, blood pressure medications, or antidepressants themselves—can sometimes trigger or worsen depressive symptoms in sensitive individuals.

What about anxiety?

Anxiety is more than just occasional worry or nervousness. It is the persistent and often overwhelming feeling of fear, dread, or unease that lingers—sometimes for hours, days, or even weeks—regardless of whether a real threat exists. While everyone experiences moments of anxiety before a big event or during times of stress, an anxiety disorder goes beyond these temporary feelings. It becomes a chronic state that interferes with a person's daily life, productivity, and sense of peace.

Anxiety can manifest in countless ways, many of them physical. You might experience:

- Restlessness or the inability to sit still

- Irritability, even in situations that wouldn't normally bother you

- Racing thoughts that won't quiet down, especially at night

- Difficulty concentrating, as your mind feels pulled in multiple directions

- Sleep disturbances, from trouble falling asleep to waking up feeling exhausted

- Tension in the body, such as tight shoulders or clenched jaw

- Digestive issues, like nausea, stomachaches, or irritable bowel symptoms

- Heart palpitations or a sensation of your chest tightening

- A constant sense of "impending doom," even when everything appears fine

These symptoms aren't imaginary or "in your head." Anxiety activates your body's stress response—what's often referred to as the "fight-or-flight" mechanism. This biological system is designed to protect us from real danger, like a wild animal chasing us. But in the case of chronic anxiety, the brain responds to perceived threats—deadlines, social situations, financial worries—as if they were immediate physical dangers.

Why do we experience anxiety?

From an evolutionary perspective, anxiety has a purpose. It sharpens our focus, raises our alertness, and helps us react quickly in the face of threat. In moderation, this is useful. But when that system is always "on," it exhausts both the body and mind. Instead of helping us survive, it begins to erode our quality of life.

For many people, anxiety stems from:

- Uncertainty about the future

- Fear of failure or rejection

- Unresolved trauma or past events

- High-pressure environments (school, work, parenting)

- Perfectionism or the fear of making mistakes

- Biological and genetic predispositions

- Substance use or withdrawal

- Hormonal changes or chronic illness

- Certain medications that heighten nervous system activity

The trap of overthinking

One hallmark of anxiety is an overactive mind that tends to latch onto worst-case scenarios. You might find yourself mentally rehearsing every possible outcome before a simple conversation or convincing yourself that something bad is about to happen—even when there's no evidence.

This "what if" loop can become exhausting:

- "What if I mess up the presentation?"

- "What if they don't like me?"

- "What if I fail?"

- "What if I never get better?"

These thoughts play on repeat, feeding the cycle of fear and self-doubt. Eventually, you may begin to avoid situations altogether—canceling plans, skipping events, or staying silent—just to feel a temporary sense of relief. Unfortunately, avoidance strengthens anxiety in the long run and shrinks your world more each day.

You are not alone

Anxiety disorders are among the most common mental health conditions in the world. Millions of people silently deal with symptoms like yours. The good news? Anxiety is treatable. With the right tools, support, and strategies, it's possible to break the cycle, calm your mind, and feel in control again.

This book will guide you through those tools—both traditional and integrative approaches—to help you understand and manage anxiety effectively.

Depression and anxiety across life stages

Mental health challenges don't discriminate by age. In children, depression can manifest as irritability, low energy, social withdrawal, or sudden academic struggles. Teenagers, already navigating identity, peer pressure, and hormonal shifts, are particularly vulnerable. Young adults may feel overwhelmed by the demands of independence and adulthood, especially without guidance or support.

For working adults, stress from career expectations, financial burdens, or parenting demands can become overwhelming. Disappointments, like unmet goals or relationship struggles, often trigger episodes of anxiety or depression. And older adults—who may face illness, isolation, or the loss of loved ones—are often overlooked when it comes to mental health, even though they may need support the most.

The vicious cycle

Depression and anxiety often work hand in hand—two emotional forces that feed and amplify one another in a relentless, exhausting loop. This cycle typically begins with worry. You start feeling anxious about something—your job, your health, your relationships, your future. Your thoughts race. You try to push them away, but they keep coming back, louder each time.

Then comes the guilt. Why can't I just stop overthinking? Why can't I calm down like everyone else? What's wrong with me? You begin to feel like a failure for having these feelings in the first place. That guilt gradually turns into sadness, hopelessness, and emotional numbness—classic symptoms of depression. You begin to withdraw. Things that once brought you joy now feel meaningless. And yet, your mind doesn't rest—it keeps worrying, now about the depression itself. What if I never feel better? What if this is who I am now?

This is the vicious cycle:

- Anxiety triggers guilt,

- Guilt leads to depression,

- Depression deepens fear and hopelessness,

- Fear reignites anxiety,

- And the loop continues.

It's like being stuck in quicksand—every thought and emotion pulling you deeper, while your energy and motivation to escape fade with time. What makes this cycle even more damaging is that it often goes unnoticed by others. From the outside, you may seem "fine." You might still go to work, smile at friends, or post pictures online. But inside, the emotional turbulence feels unbearable.

This cycle isn't just mentally draining—it takes a toll on your physical health too. Chronic anxiety and depression can disrupt your sleep, digestion, immune system, and even your cardiovascular health. Your body and brain remain in a prolonged state of stress, which makes it even harder to think clearly or take positive action.

But here's the truth—there is always a way out.

It may not be a sudden, dramatic exit. It's more often a slow climb, one small step at a time. A walk outside. A conversation with someone who listens. A breath, deep and intentional. A tiny change in routine. A moment of self-compassion. And eventually, those small choices begin to break the cycle.

Recognizing the pattern is the first step. Once you can identify how your anxiety fuels your depression—and how your depression feeds your anxiety—you can begin to interrupt that loop. This book will walk you through exactly how to do that, with tools to help you reclaim your thoughts, soothe your nervous system, and regain emotional control.

You are not broken. You are not weak. You are experiencing a very real mental health challenge that can be healed. The vicious cycle may feel powerful now, but so are you—and you're about to remember that.

How to know when it's more than just a bad day

Everyone feels low sometimes. But when symptoms persist for more than two weeks, and begin to affect your relationships, work, energy, and joy, it's time to seek help.

Common signs of depression include:

- Constant fatigue or low energy

- Loss of interest in activities you once enjoyed

- Persistent sadness or emptiness

- Changes in appetite or sleep patterns

- Difficulty concentrating or making decisions

- Feelings of worthlessness or guilt

- Thoughts of death or suicide

Common signs of anxiety include:

- Excessive worry or fear

- Restlessness or inability to relax

- Racing thoughts

- Difficulty sleeping

- Shortness of breath, sweating, or heart palpitations

- Avoidance of specific situations

Take back control

One of the most powerful truths about mental health is this: you may not be able to control what happens to you—but you can absolutely learn how to respond. That choice, however small it may seem in the moment, is a turning point. Life brings all kinds of unexpected hardships—loss, trauma, stress, conflict—but your response can determine whether these experiences define you or refine you.

Depression and anxiety often thrive in environments of fear, isolation, and misunderstanding. When we feel unsafe, disconnected, or ashamed of our struggles, those emotions gain strength. They whisper that we're alone, that no one would understand, or that something is wrong with us. But these conditions don't reflect the truth—they reflect the absence of awareness, compassion, and action.

When we bring light to our inner world—by recognizing what we're feeling, talking about it, and learning new ways to care for ourselves—the darkness begins to lose its grip. Awareness invites clarity. Compassion brings gentleness. And action moves us forward, even when it's just one step at a time.

It's also crucial to understand that mental health and physical health are deeply interconnected. Your emotional state doesn't exist in a vacuum. The brain is part of the body, and when your mind is in distress, your body often sends signals to let you know. If you find yourself constantly tired no matter how much you rest, experiencing frequent headaches, muscle tension, digestive issues, or a weakened immune response—these may be more than just random symptoms. They could be somatic expressions of unaddressed depression or anxiety.

Chronic emotional stress can dysregulate your nervous system, increase inflammation, and disrupt hormonal balance. Over time, this can lead to not just emotional fatigue, but physical burnout. You may feel like you're "falling apart," when in reality, your body is asking you to listen—to slow down, reconnect, and heal.

Unfortunately, many people spend months or even years treating only the physical symptoms—visiting multiple doctors, undergoing tests, and taking medication—without ever being asked, "How are you doing emotionally?" That question matters. And so does your honest answer.

So if you're struggling, please don't ignore what your body is trying to tell you. Depression and anxiety are not signs of weakness—they are calls for support, healing, and change. And the good news is: support exists. Healing is possible. Change is within reach.

In the chapters ahead, we'll explore not only the root causes and symptoms of these conditions, but also the practical tools, mindsets, and daily practices that can help you feel grounded, empowered, and more in control of your life again. You'll learn how to move from survival mode into a space of clarity, connection, and emotional resilience.

Because you deserve more than just "getting through" the day. You deserve to feel alive in it.

You are not alone

The World Health Organization now ranks depression as one of the leading causes of disability worldwide. Millions of people experience what you may be feeling right now. And more importantly, millions have found ways to feel better, to heal, and to reclaim their lives.

You can, too.

This book will guide you through the process of recognizing, understanding, and managing depression and anxiety. You will learn strategies that don't just mask symptoms but support lasting transformation—body, mind, and spirit.

But first, you need to know the full picture. Let's move on to the next chapter where we'll take a closer look at the specific signs and symptoms of depression—and how to recognize them before they take root.

Chapter 2

Recognizing the warning signs: how depression speaks through the mind and body

Depression rarely arrives like a thunderstorm. It tends to creep in like fog—slow, quiet, and disorienting. You don't just wake up one day overwhelmed by despair; more often, depression begins as a subtle shift: a lingering sadness, a touch of anxiety, or a feeling that something just isn't right.

This emotional descent usually starts with a thought—a worry, a memory, or a fear. Left unaddressed, this thought can spiral into anxiety. And over time, anxiety can transform into depression. That's why it's essential to recognize the early signs—in yourself and in others.

Being aware of the signals your mind and body are sending is not only empowering—it could be life-saving.

Core symptoms of depression

Below are common symptoms that may indicate depression. Keep in mind that everyone's experience is different. While you might not identify with all of these signs, if several resonate with you or persist over time, it's worth exploring them further with the help of a mental health professional.

1. Persistent feelings of hopelessness

If you begin to feel as though nothing will ever improve, or that life has lost its meaning, you may be dealing with depression. Hopelessness often pairs with helplessness—the belief that no one can help and that no effort will make a difference. These feelings can surface gradually, especially when facing prolonged stress or loss.

2. Disrupted sleep patterns

Depression commonly disrupts the body's natural sleep cycle. Some people suffer from insomnia—especially waking up too early and being unable to fall back asleep—while others experience hypersomnia, sleeping excessively and still feeling tired. Pay close attention to these patterns, as chronic sleep disruptions can worsen depressive symptoms.

3. Increased irritability or anger

Contrary to popular belief, depression doesn't always manifest as sadness. For many, it shows up as agitation, restlessness, or sudden bursts of anger. You may notice a shorter temper, lower tolerance for stress, or even episodes of lashing out—towards others or yourself. If unmanaged, these emotional outbursts can escalate and cause harm.

4. Loss of interest in previously enjoyed activities

This is one of the hallmark signs of clinical depression, known as anhedonia. When hobbies, social outings, sexual activity, or even simple pleasures like music or nature no longer bring you joy, it's a red flag. This emotional withdrawal can also lead to physical and social isolation, which only deepens the depression.

5. Low self-worth and self-criticism

Self-loathing, excessive guilt, or feelings of worthlessness are common symptoms. You may judge yourself harshly for minor mistakes, feel undeserving of love or support, or replay past failures on a loop. If your inner dialogue has become increasingly negative, it's time to take that seriously.

6. Difficulty concentrating or making decisions

If your mind feels foggy or you're struggling to focus on work, conversations, or tasks that were once easy, it could be a sign of depression. Memory lapses, indecisiveness, and a general inability to stay present are frequent complaints. These symptoms not only disrupt productivity—they fuel the cycle of frustration and emotional distress.

7. Physical pain without a clear cause

The mind and body are deeply interconnected. Depression often expresses itself physically through persistent headaches, body aches, muscle tension, and digestive problems. If your medical tests come back normal but the pain remains, it's worth considering whether emotional stress is manifesting somatically.

8. Escapist or risky behavior

Depression may drive individuals to seek relief through harmful distractions. This includes substance abuse, reckless driving, binge eating, compulsive spending, gambling, or even overworking. These behaviors are attempts to numb emotional pain—but they often lead to deeper emotional turmoil and addiction if left unchecked.

9. Fatigue and lack of energy

Even without doing much, a depressed person often feels physically drained. The exhaustion isn't just tiredness—it's a sense of heaviness in the body and soul. Tasks that once took five minutes may feel insurmountable. This loss of motivation isn't laziness—it's a symptom of an overwhelmed nervous system.

10. Appetite and weight changes

Both significant weight loss and weight gain can be signs of depression. Some individuals experience a sharp decline in appetite, while others turn to food for comfort. These shifts can cause body image issues, shame, and further emotional distress, deepening the cycle of depression.

Depression is a process—so is healing

Depression doesn't announce itself—it unfolds. That's why self-awareness is key. If you can recognize these symptoms early, you have a better chance of intervening before they take root. The same goes for supporting a loved one: if you notice these signs in someone close to you, don't ignore them. Compassionate presence and gentle conversation can make a world of difference.

The signs of depression are not just emotional—they are physiological, cognitive, and behavioral. If left unchecked, these symptoms can lead to chronic stress, increased anxiety, and a cascade of health complications, including weakened immunity, sleep disorders, and heart disease.

This chapter was created to help you name what you're feeling. In naming, you gain power. In understanding, you find options. In acknowledgment, you open the door to healing.

What happens if symptoms are ignored?

Unchecked symptoms of depression don't just linger quietly in the background—they tend to intensify and spread, affecting every area of life. What may begin as fatigue or sadness can deepen into emotional numbness, making it difficult to feel anything at all, even joy or love. As the emotional void grows, some people turn to coping mechanisms like alcohol, drugs, overeating, or compulsive behaviors—temporary escapes that often create new problems rather than solve existing ones.

In more severe cases, these unchecked symptoms may lead to thoughts of self-harm or suicide. Depression distorts perception, convincing the mind that nothing will ever get better, that one's pain is permanent and unfixable. This is a dangerous illusion—because depression is treatable, and recovery is not only possible, it is likely with the right tools and support.

Ignoring the signs, however, allows the condition to take deeper root. Over time, neural pathways in the brain reinforce these negative emotional patterns, making it more difficult to shift out of them. The longer depression goes unaddressed, the more entrenched it becomes—not because you are weak or broken, but because the brain is simply following the path it has practiced most often.

That's why this chapter—and this book—aren't here to alarm you, but to equip you. Awareness is power. When you can name what you're going through, you create space for healing. Early recognition gives you the opportunity to interrupt the spiral and begin the upward journey.

In the next chapter, we'll explore what happens when depression fully sets in—emotionally, physically, neurologically—and how that affects your overall wellbeing. Most importantly, we'll begin introducing science-backed tools and holistic practices to help you gently but powerfully restore your mind, body, and spirit.

Your story is not over. This moment, right now, is part of your turning point. Let's keep moving forward—together.

Understanding the early symptoms of depression is not just helpful—it's essential. In a world that often tells us to push through pain, smile through struggle, and "toughen up," it can be incredibly easy to miss or dismiss the signs your body and mind are trying to send you.

Cultural expectations, social roles, religious beliefs, and generational conditioning often reward endurance and discourage vulnerability. We are taught to be strong, resilient, productive. To keep going no matter what. And while there is power in perseverance, there is also danger in silence.

Ignoring subtle shifts in mood, energy, appetite, motivation, or thought patterns simply because "others have it worse" or "you should be grateful" leads to one painful outcome: the illness settles in deeper. Depression doesn't always arrive with dramatic breakdowns or visible tears. Sometimes, it shows up quietly—through fatigue, irritability, disinterest in things you used to love, or a constant sense of heaviness that you can't explain. And when you don't acknowledge those signs, they grow.

Society often glorifies those who seem to "have it all together," but here's the truth: people can look happy and be deeply unwell. Smiles can be masks. Success can coexist with emptiness. Someone can be leading meetings, raising children, posting joyful moments on social media—and still cry in the shower or feel hollow inside. Depression wears many disguises, and that's why awareness matters so much.

Your internal experience is valid, even if it doesn't match the expectations of your external world. Listening to yourself—really listening—is an act of self-preservation. Your body speaks in whispers before it screams, and the earlier you catch those whispers, the more gently you can heal.

So please don't wait until everything falls apart to take your mental health seriously. Don't let the pressure to "be fine" rob you of your chance to truly be well. The brave thing isn't pretending it's okay—it's admitting when it's not, and choosing to do something about it.

Because depression thrives in silence, but healing begins with awareness.

Chapter 3

When the mind hurts, the body follows

The health effects of depression

Understanding what depression is and recognizing its symptoms is only the beginning. Now that you've begun to identify its presence in your life or the life of someone you love, it's time to look deeper—at what depression actually does to your health.

Depression is not "just in your head." It's not something you can simply snap out of. It's a condition with real, measurable effects on your physical, emotional, and neurological well-being. Left unchecked, depression begins to erode the body from within, quietly and persistently, often before you even realize the damage.

The truth is: depression is a whole-body illness. Its effects ripple through every system in your body, amplifying other medical conditions and sometimes masking itself as purely physical ailments. That's why it's crucial to understand what's really happening inside you—because awareness is power, and power is the first step toward healing.

1. Higher risk of heart disease

People living with depression are significantly more likely to experience cardiovascular problems, including heart attacks and strokes. Why? Because depression triggers chronic stress responses in the body—releasing excess cortisol, elevating blood pressure, and increasing inflammation.

When these internal stress chemicals are always "on," your heart and blood vessels are under constant pressure. Depression doesn't just weigh down your spirit—it physically weighs down your cardiovascular system too.

2. Weight fluctuations and disordered Eating

Depression alters your appetite. For some, it causes emotional eating or bingeing in search of comfort. For others, it suppresses the desire to eat entirely. The result? Rapid weight gain or dangerous weight loss—both of which carry health risks like diabetes, high cholesterol, and weakened immunity.

And beyond the physical impact, the emotional toll of body image issues—shame, insecurity, guilt—only deepens the depressive spiral.

3. Insomnia and disturbed sleep

When your mind can't rest, your body won't either. Depression and anxiety often disrupt sleep in the form of insomnia, racing thoughts, or waking up too early and being unable to fall back asleep.

Sleep deprivation affects concentration, emotional regulation, and immune function. The lack of rest becomes a feedback loop—less sleep worsens depression, which leads to even less sleep.

4. Persistent fatigue and energy drain

Chronic exhaustion is one of the most common symptoms of depression. It's not the kind of tiredness that sleep fixes—it's a heavy, unrelenting fatigue that makes even basic daily tasks feel monumental. You may feel like your body is moving through molasses, your motivation gone, and your spark dulled.

Fatigue caused by depression is both physical and emotional, and it can be completely disabling without intervention.

5. Weakened immune system

Prolonged depression has a suppressive effect on your immune system, leaving you vulnerable to frequent colds, infections, and slower recovery from illness. Stress hormones like cortisol interfere with your body's ability to fight disease.

If you find yourself getting sick more often than usual, depression may be silently compromising your immune defenses.

6. Increased sensitivity to pain

One of the lesser-known effects of depression is that it amplifies physical pain. People suffering from depression often report more intense headaches, joint pain, muscle aches, and back pain—yet medication offers little relief. That's because the brain's ability to regulate pain perception is altered by mood disorders.

This is why treating the underlying depression often reduces physical discomfort as well.

7. Constricted blood vessels and cardiovascular strain

Depression can lead to vasoconstriction—the narrowing of blood vessels—which raises blood pressure and puts additional strain on the heart. Over time, this can lead to serious complications like hypertension and heart disease. Mental tension becomes physical tension. The body mirrors the mind's distress.

8. Suicidal ideation and self-harm

This is the most dangerous effect of untreated depression. When depression becomes overwhelming, it can lead to persistent thoughts of death, hopelessness, and suicide. People in this state often feel like they're a burden, like nothing will ever change, or that the pain will never end.

If you or someone you know is experiencing suicidal thoughts, it is vital to seek help immediately. Suicide is a permanent solution to a temporary pain—and there is always a path back to light, even if you can't see it in the moment.

9. Memory loss and cognitive decline

Depression affects the brain's ability to process information, focus, and store memory. You may find yourself forgetting things, unable to concentrate, or struggling to make decisions. In older adults, long-term depression has even been linked to an increased risk of dementia and Alzheimer's disease.

10. Chronic headaches and neurological stress

When your brain is under constant emotional stress, your nervous system suffers. Depression often manifests as chronic tension headaches or migraines, which become a vicious cycle of pain and psychological strain. These headaches are not merely physical—they're neurological distress signals from a mind in pain.

The hidden cost of depression

Perhaps the most dangerous thing about depression is its invisibility.

It can disguise itself behind perfectly curated smiles, productive schedules, and everyday routines. People learn to wear masks—at work, with friends, even with family. They laugh on cue, answer emails, attend meetings, help others... all while crumbling inside. They become masters of disguise, concealing their pain in plain sight. They say "I'm fine" not because they are, but because they've convinced themselves they have to be.

But the body knows the truth. It absorbs every emotional blow. Every silent scream lodged in the chest. Every tear never cried. Every fear buried deep to avoid judgment.

Over time, the toll becomes too much. Like a dam under pressure, it eventually cracks. Sometimes it shows up in the form of illness. Other times, in exhaustion, breakdowns, or complete emotional shutdown.

This is why we must talk about depression—not just in clinical terms, but in human ones. Because it doesn't always look like sadness. Sometimes, it looks like overachievement. Sometimes, it looks like irritability, or withdrawal, or chronic fatigue. Sometimes, it looks like the strongest person you know falling apart when no one's watching.

Depression is not weakness. It's not a character flaw. It's not something that can be "snapped out of." And it is certainly not something to be ashamed of.

It is a medical condition—a disorder of the brain, emotions, and body—that deserves the same compassion and treatment as any other illness.

When society tells you to toughen up, when your culture says "we don't talk about this," when your inner critic whispers that you're being dramatic—remember this:

You are not broken. You are human. And help is not just available—it is necessary, and you deserve it.

Now that you understand how deeply depression can affect not just your mood, but your physical and mental well-being, the next step is crucial. It's time to explore how to reverse the damage—one gentle, conscious step at a time.

Science-backed tools. Therapeutic practices. Small, powerful habits. Shifts in your inner dialogue. Support systems that hold space for your healing.

You don't have to do it all at once. You just have to begin.

Because the sooner you address the root, the sooner you'll feel the light returning.

And even if it feels far away now, healing is always within reach.

Chapter 4

10 reseach-backed strategies to overcome depression and reclaim your life

We've talked about what depression is, the symptoms it brings, and how it affects every corner of your life. But now we arrive at what may be the most important part of your journey: learning how to fight back.

This chapter is not a promise of overnight transformation—but a practical guide to help you take the first steps out of darkness. It combines scientific findings, proven therapeutic approaches, and the wisdom of countless people who've fought depression and found relief.

The goal here is not perfection—it's progress. These are not magic tricks or quick fixes. They are sustainable practices that gradually rewire your brain, restore emotional balance, and help you reclaim your power.

Let's get into the ten most effective tools to manage and reduce depression symptoms:

1. Recognize and silence your inner critic

One of the most powerful first steps is to become aware of the internal dialogue that fuels depression. Negative self-talk—blaming yourself, replaying failures, judging your emotions—acts like poison to your mental health.

Psychologists call this pattern "cognitive distortion," and it's a hallmark of depression. These distorted thoughts aren't truths—they're mental habits. Using techniques from cognitive behavioral therapy (CBT), you can learn to identify these thought traps, challenge them, and begin to replace them with more compassionate, realistic beliefs.

It's important to understand that we all carry what some call "demons" inside us—not literal monsters, but emotional wounds, unresolved fears, shame, anger, sadness. These parts of us often show up as harsh inner voices, and our instinct is to fight them off or suppress them. But healing isn't about waging war with yourself. It's about learning how to coexist with all parts of you, even the painful ones.

These "demons" can be managed, softened, and even silenced—not through denial, but through understanding and compassion. You don't have to let them drive your decisions or define your identity.

☐ **What helps:** Begin journaling your negative thoughts. When one arises, write it down and respond as if you're comforting a friend. Ask yourself: "Would I say this to someone I love?" If the answer is no, you shouldn't say it to yourself.

Also, consider distancing yourself—emotionally or physically—from people who reinforce your self-doubt, invalidate your pain, or feed your inner critic. You don't need people in your life who echo the voices you're trying to quiet.

Protect your peace. Befriend your mind. And remember: your thoughts are not facts—they are patterns. And patterns can be rewritten.

2. Don't isolate—stay connected

Depression urges you to withdraw from others, convincing you that you're a burden, that no one would understand, or that you're better off alone. But isolation doesn't protect you—it amplifies the pain. It creates an echo chamber where negative thoughts grow louder and hope feels more distant.

Even when it's uncomfortable or feels exhausting, making the effort to stay connected is a powerful act of self-care. You don't need to have the perfect words or a big breakthrough—just being around someone who listens without judgment can create space for healing. Sometimes, being seen and heard is enough to start mending what feels broken.

Human connection isn't just emotional—it's biological. Studies show that when we engage in safe, empathetic conversation, our brain releases oxytocin, the bonding hormone. Oxytocin not only strengthens emotional closeness but also reduces cortisol, the stress hormone. This physiological response creates a sense of calm and safety, helping your nervous system return to balance. In other words, connection is literally medicine for the mind.

You don't have to be surrounded by crowds. One genuine, supportive relationship can be more healing than a hundred shallow ones. Whether it's a friend, a relative, a therapist, or even a support group online, what matters most is finding someone who listens and holds space for you to simply be.

☐ **What helps:**

- Reach out to one trusted person—someone who cares and doesn't try to "fix" you but simply stays present.

- Set a manageable goal: a weekly phone call, a walk, a coffee meetup, or even a text exchange. Ten minutes of real connection can interrupt the spiral of isolation.

- If you're unsure who to reach out to, consider joining a support group or online forum for people dealing with depression. Sometimes, strangers walking the same path offer unexpected comfort.

Connection doesn't cure everything, but it reminds you that you're not alone. And when you're struggling in the dark, even one light can help guide you home.

3. Be compassionate with yourself

Depression is not your fault. You didn't choose it. It's not a sign of weakness, laziness, or failure. And it certainly doesn't define who you are.

Yet so many people silently carry the weight of shame, as if they *should* be able to snap out of it, as if asking for help means they're broken. This shame becomes an invisible cage—one that keeps you stuck, doubting yourself, and reinforcing the very pain you're trying to escape.

But here's a liberating truth: you are not your symptoms. You are a human being experiencing a very real, very valid condition—one that affects millions and has deep emotional, physiological, and neurological roots.

That's why *practicing self-compassion* isn't just comforting advice—it's a therapeutic tool backed by science. According to neuroscience research, when you treat yourself with warmth and empathy instead of criticism, your brain activates the parasympathetic nervous system—your body's rest-and-heal mode. This response releases oxytocin and other calming neurochemicals, reducing stress, quieting the inner critic, and making room for healing.

Self-compassion doesn't mean denying your pain or pretending everything is okay. It means saying: *"This is hard, and I'm hurting—but I still deserve love, support, and care."*

In fact, studies have shown that self-compassion is strongly associated with decreased levels of anxiety and depression, and increased resilience, motivation, and emotional wellbeing.

☐ **What helps:**

- When you feel overwhelmed, try this simple mantra: *"This is difficult, but I am doing the best I can. I am allowed to feel this. I deserve kindness."*

- Write a compassionate letter to yourself, the way you would to a friend going through the same struggle.

- Practice gentle touch—like placing your hand over your heart—and breathing deeply. This activates the vagus nerve and helps calm the mind-body stress response.

- Remember: being kind to yourself in hard moments is not weakness—it's emotional strength in its truest form.

You are worthy of love and care—not *despite* your pain, but *because* you are human**.** Learning to treat yourself with the same grace you'd extend to someone you love is one of the most powerful steps toward healing.

4. Add joy—even if you don't feel it

Pleasure may feel out of reach when you're depressed—but it still matters.

One of the cruel tricks of depression is that it dulls your ability to feel joy. Things that used to excite you now feel meaningless or effortful. You might think, *What's the point?* or *I'll never enjoy that again.* But this is not the truth of who you are—it's a symptom. And symptoms can shift.

This is where Behavioral Activation Therapy comes in. It's a well-studied, evidence-based strategy used in cognitive behavioral therapy (CBT) that works by gently nudging you back into life—not by waiting for motivation, but by creating it through action.

The concept is simple but powerful: you don't have to wait until you feel better to start doing better**.** In fact, acting *before* you feel like it can help break the cycle of avoidance and emotional numbness. Even small actions—when repeated—can send a signal to your brain that life is still worth engaging with.

☐ **What helps:**

- Schedule one small enjoyable thing every day, even if it feels silly or forced at first. This could be:

    ◦ Listening to a favorite song

    ◦ Watching a funny video or comedy show

    ◦ Taking a short walk in nature

    ◦ Doing a creative hobby (drawing, cooking, dancing)

    ◦ Lighting a candle and sitting in silence

    ◦ Petting a dog or cat

    ◦ Smelling essential oils or flowers

These moments may seem insignificant, but they help rewire your brain, activating reward circuits and slowly rebuilding your capacity for pleasure and connection. Over time, these small sparks can become the foundation for real, lasting change.

Even laughter—especially laughter—has therapeutic benefits. It reduces stress hormones, increases endorphins, and helps you feel more connected to the present moment.

Think of these activities as "emotional vitamins." You might not feel their full effect right away, but with consistent use, they nourish your nervous system and remind your mind: *joy is still possible.*

You don't need to feel joy to begin seeking it. You only need to take one step toward it—and trust that the feeling may follow.

5. Move your body

Exercise is one of the most studied and powerful tools for managing depression.

When you're struggling with depression, moving your body can feel like the last thing you want to do. But science shows that physical activity can be just as effective as medication or therapy in reducing symptoms of mild to moderate depression. The reason? Movement activates your brain's natural feel-good chemicals—serotonin, dopamine, and endorphins—which help regulate mood, motivation, focus, and emotional resilience.

Regular exercise also lowers levels of cortisol, the stress hormone that tends to be elevated in people with depression and anxiety. It improves sleep quality, energy levels, and self-esteem, creating a positive feedback loop that supports long-term emotional well-being.

You don't have to run a marathon or spend hours at the gym. In fact, gentle, consistent movement can be just as healing—and far more sustainable.

□ **What helps:**

- Start small. Even 20 minutes of brisk walking a day has been shown to significantly improve mood and reduce anxiety.

- Focus on movement you enjoy. That could mean:

  - Yoga or tai chi

  - Dancing in your living room

  - Swimming or cycling

  - Stretching while listening to music

  - Nature walks or gardening

The key is consistency, not intensity. Depression often thrives on stagnation—physically and emotionally. Movement reminds your body that you are alive, capable, and in motion.

Think of movement as a daily signal to your brain: *I am choosing life. I am reclaiming control.*

If possible, try exercising outdoors. Natural light and fresh air further support your mental health by regulating your circadian rhythm and increasing vitamin D levels, both of which are often disrupted in people with depression.

You don't have to "feel like it" to start. Just move a little. Breathe. Stretch. Walk. Repeat. The shift begins there.

6. Practice daily gratitude

Gratitude physically rewires your brain.

Gratitude isn't just a feel-good practice—it's a powerful tool with measurable effects on the brain. Studies using functional MRI scans have shown that people who regularly engage in gratitude practices—like journaling or writing thank-you notes—experience increased activity in the prefrontal cortex, the region of the brain involved in empathy, emotional regulation, decision-making, and long-term wellbeing.

In other words, the more you practice gratitude, the more your brain becomes wired to experience joy, hope, and connection.

When you're depressed, your mind is trained to notice what's wrong. Gratitude gently retrains the brain to look for what's right—even in difficult moments. This doesn't mean ignoring pain or pretending everything is okay; it means making space for light to coexist with darkness.

Gratitude also helps reduce the effects of cortisol (the stress hormone) and boosts dopamine and serotonin, creating a neurochemical environment that supports healing and emotional resilience.

□ **What helps:**

- **Write down three things you're grateful for every day.** They don't have to be big. A warm cup of tea. A text from a friend. A moment of silence.

- **Be specific.** "I'm grateful for the way the sunlight came through the window this morning." Specificity helps your brain anchor the experience.

- **Say thank you more often.** Even silently. Thank your body for carrying you through the day. Thank your past self for surviving hard things.

- **Return to your gratitude list when you feel low.** It's a map back to hope.

Gratitude doesn't erase pain—it expands your capacity to hold both beauty and sorrow.

Over time, these small acts build a stronger emotional foundation. You're not just writing words—you're changing the lens through which your brain sees the world.

7. Acknowledge and release anger

Sometimes depression is a mask for unresolved anger.

Not all depression comes from sadness. In fact, in many cases, it is suppressed anger—the kind that hasn't found a voice or an outlet. You might be angry at someone who hurt you, at a situation that feels unfair, or even at yourself for perceived mistakes or missed opportunities.

When anger doesn't have a safe way to express itself, it often turns inward. That's when it begins to show up as self-criticism, shame, guilt, or deep sadness. Over time, that emotional tension builds up in the body, leading to chronic fatigue, tight muscles, digestive issues, or even auto-immune flares.

This kind of repressed emotional energy doesn't just go away—it leaks out in unexpected ways: irritability, emotional numbness, or a sense of helplessness that fuels depression.

☐ **What helps:**

- **Name the anger without judgment.** Anger is not wrong. It's an emotion that often points to a boundary being crossed or a need going unmet.

- **Journal honestly.** Let the words come out raw. Write letters you don't send. Say what you really feel on the page.

- **Try expressive outlets.** Punch a pillow. Paint with bold strokes. Shout into a towel. Go for a fast walk or do an intense workout. Use your body to release what your words can't say.

- **Work with a therapist.** A trained professional can help you untangle the roots of anger and process it safely, especially if it's linked to trauma.

- **Practice self-forgiveness.** If you're angry at yourself, remind yourself that you were doing the best you could with what you had at the time.

Anger is not your enemy. Unacknowledged anger is. When you give anger a healthy voice, it loses its power to sabotage your peace.

Remember: Healing doesn't come from silence—it comes from release. Let your anger speak. Then, guide it into transformation.

8. Help others

Helping others can help you heal.

When you're deep in depression, your world often narrows. It becomes hard to see beyond your own pain, and even the smallest tasks can feel overwhelming. But stepping outside of your internal world—even for a short moment—to help someone else can create a powerful shift.

Studies have shown that acts of kindness and volunteering can reduce symptoms of depression and anxiety, increase feelings of connection, and boost self-esteem. This is not just emotional—it's neurological. Helping others activates reward pathways in the brain, releasing oxytocin, dopamine, and serotonin—the same feel-good chemicals targeted by antidepressants.

When you offer compassion, empathy, and service, your mind begins to remember: *you still matter*. You have something to give. You have value that isn't defined by your struggles.

☐ **What helps:**

- **Start small.** You don't have to join a big organization. Helping a neighbor, texting someone going through a hard time, or offering to walk a friend's dog can make a difference.

- **Volunteer where your heart is.** Whether it's a local animal shelter, a food bank, a hospital, or a youth program, giving your time to something that aligns with your values helps reconnect you with meaning and purpose.

- **Practice micro-kindness.** Smile at a stranger. Hold the door. Leave a kind note. These tiny moments of human connection add up—and they help you feel like you're part of something larger than yourself.

- **Reflect on the impact.** After an act of service, take a moment to sit with how it made you feel. Journaling about the experience can reinforce those positive emotional associations.

Volunteering isn't about fixing the world. It's about reclaiming your place in it.

When you contribute to others' wellbeing, you remind yourself that you're not broken—you're still powerful, capable, and needed. Sometimes, helping others is the first step to remembering how to help yourself.

9. Unplug from comparison

Social media isn't reality—it's a highlight reel.

When you're already feeling vulnerable, anxious, or low, scrolling through curated images of other people's "perfect lives" can be emotionally damaging. Social media platforms often present a distorted reality: flawless bodies, smiling faces, dream vacations, loving relationships. But what you're seeing is not the full story—it's the version people *choose* to show.

Behind every filtered photo is a human being with struggles, insecurities, and pain—just like you.

For someone battling depression or anxiety, social media can amplify feelings of inadequacy, loneliness, and self-doubt. You might find yourself comparing your low moments to someone else's best moments, and that's not a fair comparison. It's like comparing your behind-the-scenes footage to someone else's movie trailer.

In fact, research has shown that excessive social media use is linked to higher rates of depression, anxiety, sleep disturbances, and poor body image—especially among teens and young adults. Social comparison is powerful, and when it's repeated daily, it begins to rewire your brain toward chronic dissatisfaction.

□ **What helps:**

- **Take breaks.** Set time limits for apps, or consider a digital detox. Even a 24-hour break can help reset your mindset.

- **Curate your feed intentionally.** Follow people who inspire, uplift, educate, or show real vulnerability—not just polished perfection.

- **Mute or unfollow accounts that trigger comparison or self-judgment.** You have every right to protect your mental space.

- **Replace screen time with soul time.** Swap 15 minutes of scrolling for journaling, listening to music, or stepping outside.

- **Remind yourself: real life isn't always Instagrammable.** Most people don't post about their breakdowns, heartbreaks, or therapy sessions. But they're happening—even if you don't see them.

You're not behind. You're not failing. You're just seeing the *edited* version of other people's lives.

Don't let someone else's digital illusion rob you of your self-worth. Choose to consume content that reminds you of your own strength, your real beauty, and your infinite potential—as you are.

10. Seek professional help

You are not alone—and you do not have to figure this out alone.

Depression can feel like a solitary battle, but millions of people are walking through similar struggles—and many have found their way back to hope with the right help. You don't need to have all the answers. You don't even need to know where to begin. What matters is your willingness to reach out.

Therapy is one of the most effective tools for overcoming depression. It offers more than just someone to talk to—it's a structured, evidence-based process that helps you untangle the patterns that keep you stuck and teaches you how to respond in healthier, more empowered ways.

Among the most researched and effective methods are:

- **Cognitive Behavioral Therapy (CBT):** Helps you recognize and change negative thought patterns and behaviors.

- **Interpersonal Therapy (IPT):** Focuses on your relationships and how they influence your mood.

- **Psychodynamic Therapy:** Explores deeper emotional roots and unresolved conflicts.

- **Acceptance and Commitment Therapy (ACT):** Teaches mindfulness and emotional flexibility, especially for chronic depression.

For some, therapy alone is enough. For others, especially in moderate to severe depression, medication can be life-saving. Antidepressants like SSRIs (Selective Serotonin Reuptake Inhibitors) and SNRIs (Serotonin-Norepinephrine Reuptake Inhibitors) work by adjusting brain chemistry to support emotional stability, clarity, and energy. These medications don't "numb" you—they create a more level playing field so you can begin to heal.

Many people fear taking medication due to stigma or misunderstanding. But depression is not a weakness of character—it is a medical condition, and just like high blood pressure or diabetes, it sometimes requires pharmaceutical support.

And here's something important to remember:

Why go through all of this alone when there are people who have dedicated their lives to understanding and treating depression? Mental health professionals—therapists, psychiatrists, researchers—spend years studying how to help you heal. You are not a burden for needing support. In fact, asking for help is one of the most courageous steps you can take.

☐ **What helps:**

- **Find a licensed therapist**—someone trained to walk with you through this process.

- **Online therapy platforms** like *BetterHelp*, *Talkspace*, and *Open Path Collective* offer convenient, affordable options from home.

- **Speak with a psychiatrist or primary care provider** about whether medication may help support your recovery.

- **Explore sliding scale clinics** if cost is a concern—many communities offer free or low-cost services.

Healing doesn't mean doing it all on your own.It means allowing yourself to be supported.You deserve the right care. You deserve relief. You deserve to feel better.

Final thoughts

The path out of depression is not linear. There will be days when you feel a glimmer of hope and clarity—days when you manage to get out of bed, go for a walk, or smile at something small. These are victories. There will also be days when the weight returns, and it feels like you're back at square one. That's okay too. Healing is not about perfection. It's about persistence.

Progress isn't always visible, but it's happening. Even when you don't feel like you're moving forward, every effort—no matter how small—is a message to your brain that you still care. That you are still here. That you are still trying. And that matters more than you know.

Whether you've chosen to try one tool from this chapter or committed to practicing all ten, know this: you are not broken. You are becoming. You are in the process of learning to live again. Of choosing yourself. Of building something new from the inside out.

This isn't just about managing symptoms—it's about reclaiming your life.

With each conscious breath, with each act of self-kindness, with each choice to stay, you're rewriting your story—not defined by pain, but by strength, awareness, and choice.

And you don't have to do it perfectly. You just have to keep going.

In the next chapter, we'll explore the power of mindset and how your thoughts shape your reality. You'll learn how to identify mental patterns that fuel suffering—and how to rewire them to support healing, growth, and emotional resilience.

Remember: You are not alone in this. You are not weak. And you are stronger than you think. This is not the end of your story—it's the beginning of your transformation.

Chapter 5
Training your mind for resilience

T raining your mind for resilience: how mental habits shape your emotional health
Everything you feel—every emotion, every reaction, every internal struggle—stems from your mind. Whether you wake up feeling empowered or defeated, optimistic or overwhelmed, it often starts with the beliefs and narratives you hold inside. That's why mental health professionals and neuroscientists agree: true healing requires mental training—not just positive thinking, but a complete shift in how you process and respond to life.

You can't simply think your way out of depression. But you can train your mind to stop reinforcing the same patterns that keep you stuck.

In this chapter, you'll learn how to educate your mind to become a place of stability, strength, and clarity. Think of it like building a mental fortress—one that doesn't allow every fear or intrusive thought to invade and take control. When your mind is properly trained, the rest of your life can begin to realign.

How depression begins in the mind

If you reflect on your own experience with anxiety or depression, you may be able to trace it back to a moment—a thought, a headline, a conversation, or a feeling—that took root. It might have been subtle, like a whisper of worry that spiraled into sleepless nights. Or a passing fear that grew into a full sense of despair.

For example, an entrepreneur might read a grim forecast about the economy. At first, it's just a concern. But then come the thoughts:"What if my business fails?""What if I lose everything?""How will I provide for my family?"

These are not just thoughts. They are mental scripts—and the brain, especially when overwhelmed, repeats them like background music. The more the thoughts repeat, the more the body reacts with stress, tension, and anxiety. Left unchecked, these thoughts can build an inner environment where depression thrives.

But here's the good news: You are not powerless against your thoughts.The mind can be trained. And when you train it well, it becomes your ally—not your enemy.

6 proven strategies to educate and strengthen the mind

1. Feed your mind intentionally

Your brain is not a passive observer—it's an active filter, constantly absorbing and processing everything around you. Every conversation you engage in, every news story you scroll past, every podcast you listen to, and even the background noise playing while you cook or drive is shaping your internal world.

This constant intake of information has a powerful effect on your mood, focus, and your ability to regulate emotions and cope with stress. If you're surrounded by negativity—whether it's fear-based news, toxic online debates, or pessimistic people—your brain begins to mirror that tone. It starts to anticipate threats, dwell on problems, and magnify what's going wrong.

Neuroscience has shown that the brain responds to repeated messages by reinforcing those pathways. If you're constantly exposed to information that's discouraging or chaotic, your brain wires itself for fear and anxiety. On the other hand, exposure to inspiring, healing, and empowering messages can activate the brain's reward centers, increase motivation, and even promote neuroplasticity—the ability to adapt and grow new thought patterns.

□What helps:

Start treating your attention like your most valuable asset—because it is. Just as you wouldn't eat spoiled food, don't consume content that poisons your peace.

- Read books that expand your perspective, nurture hope, and teach resilience.

- Follow mental health professionals and creators who share tools, not just trauma.

- Listen to podcasts rooted in neuroscience, mindfulness, and practical healing strategies.

- Take breaks from the news and social media when needed, and don't be afraid to unfollow anything that leaves you feeling heavy or inferior.

- Surround yourself with voices—in person and online—that remind you of your worth, not your shortcomings.

What you feed your mind shapes how it thinks, what it focuses on, and how it responds to life. Make it a daily habit to give your brain something healing to hold onto.

2. Consciously reframe negative thoughts

The goal is not to "eliminate" all negative thoughts—that's not only impossible, but also unnecessary. Negative thoughts are a natural part of the human experience. They arise from fear, past experiences, cultural conditioning, and even protective instincts. The real challenge is not letting those thoughts define you or dictate your reality.

Trying to suppress every negative thought can backfire and create more tension. Instead, the goal is to build awareness—to notice those thoughts when they arise, question their validity, and consciously replace them with more empowering alternatives.

This is the essence of cognitive restructuring, a cornerstone of Cognitive Behavioral Therapy (CBT)—a highly effective, evidence-based approach for treating depression, anxiety, and self-defeating patterns. The practice trains your brain to challenge irrational beliefs and reinforce more balanced, self-supportive thinking.

□What helps:

When you catch yourself thinking something like:

"I'm not good enough.""Nothing ever works out for me.""I always fail."

Pause and ask yourself:

- "Where did that thought come from?"(Was it from a past experience? Someone else's criticism? A fear of being judged?)

- "Is this thought a fact, or is it just a fear or assumption?"(Often, you'll realize it's not grounded in truth.)

Then, without judgment, replace it with a thought that reflects reality and growth, like:

"I'm learning, and that counts.""It's okay to stumble—I've overcome hard things before.""I may not feel strong now, but I am taking steps toward healing."

It's not about toxic positivity or denying hardship. It's about giving yourself a fighting chance to shift the narrative from helplessness to hope.

Practicing this daily can help rewire your neural pathways, reduce rumination, and gradually lift the fog of depression. You're not just thinking differently—you're healing your brain from the inside out.

3. Be at peace with imperfection

We all live with internal "demons"—those shadowy parts of ourselves that include uncomfortable emotions, past regrets, trauma, anger, shame, guilt, self-doubt, and insecurities. These aren't flaws in your character—they're part of being human. But many people make the mistake of spending their lives fighting these inner experiences, trying to suppress or avoid them at all costs. The problem is, what we resist tends to persist.

By constantly pushing these emotions away, we give them more power in the background of our minds. They start to shape our thoughts, reactions, and behaviors in subtle ways. The fight becomes exhausting, and often, depression or anxiety is the result of this long, internal battle.

But what if, instead of fighting them, you learned to coexist with them?

What if you stopped trying to "win" and instead focused on listening, understanding, and softening the grip of these internal voices?

□What helps:

Rather than running from uncomfortable emotions, try acknowledging them mindfully and with compassion.

Mindfulness-based practices and Acceptance and Commitment Therapy (ACT) suggest a radically different approach:

"Hello, fear. I see you're here again.""I recognize sadness. You've been around before.""Self-doubt, I hear what you're saying—but I'm still going to try."

By naming these feelings and creating space for them without judgment, you teach your brain and nervous system something powerful: that discomfort is not dangerous—it's manageable and temporary.

This shift reduces the intensity of emotions over time. You stop fueling the internal war, and instead, develop an inner peace that isn't dependent on feeling "perfect" or "happy" all the time.

In fact, your ability **to** sit with your emotions rather than run from them is one of the greatest forms of strength and emotional resilience you can build.

4. Be aware of your thought patterns

Most people aren't fully aware of what their mind is doing throughout the day. Thoughts come and go automatically, shaped by habit, past experiences, fears, and societal influences. Without conscious awareness, these thoughts can quietly shape your beliefs, mood, and behaviors—often in ways that are self-sabotaging. Destructive thoughts can take root like weeds in an unguarded garden, growing stronger the longer they go unexamined.

When you're not aware of your thinking patterns, your mind can fall into autopilot: reliving past mistakes, catastrophizing the future, or telling yourself you're not enough. This unconscious mental chatter feeds anxiety, depression, and low self-esteem—and most of the time, it's happening beneath your awareness.

But here's the good news: you can train your mind to observe itself. This skill is called meta-cognition—the ability to think about your thinking—and it's a powerful tool for mental clarity and emotional resilience.

□What helps:

Start by practicing gentle self-inquiry when a thought or belief arises. Instead of immediately accepting it as truth, pause and ask:

- "Where is this thought leading me?"

- "Is it helping me grow or holding me back?"

- "Would I believe this if someone else said it about me?"

- "Is this fact or just fear?"

By stepping into the role of the observer, you create space between you and your thoughts. That space is where choice lives. You begin to see that you are not your thoughts—you are the awareness behind them.

You can choose which thoughts to water and which to release. You can replace destructive narratives with compassionate and empowering ones. And over time, with consistent practice, you can rewire your brain to support your healing and growth.

This is the essence of mental mastery—not forcing your mind to be positive all the time, but learning to navigate it with curiosity, courage, and intention.

5. Create a mental hygiene routine

Just like physical hygiene requires daily care, so does your mental wellbeing. You wouldn't skip brushing your teeth—why skip clearing your mind?
  □ What helps:
  - Start and end your day with mental resets: gratitude journaling, affirmations, or guided meditations.

  - Avoid doom-scrolling or overstimulation before bed.

  - Reflect on your thought patterns at night and consciously choose a peaceful, empowering image or phrase to sleep on. Your brain continues processing while you rest—give it something nourishing.

6. Build resilience through consistency

Mental training: a lifelong practice for resilience and growth.

Mental training is not a one-time fix—it's not a single meditation, a temporary motivational quote, or a week of journaling. It's a daily discipline, just like brushing your teeth or nourishing your body. Every day, your brain is exposed to new inputs: news, conversations, stress, loss, pressure, comparison, change. Some of those inputs uplift you. Others can trigger anxiety, fear, or self-doubt.

That's why mental education and emotional resilience must be ongoing. Just as you wouldn't expect to stay physically fit after one gym session, you can't expect lasting emotional stability without consistent effort.

DEPRESSION, ARE YOU OK?   41

Your thoughts create mental habits. If those habits are not tended to, they default to survival mode—overthinking, catastrophizing, self-criticism. But with intentional mental training, you can create new default patterns rooted in strength, presence, and self-trust.

▢What helps:

- Be consistent with your tools. Whether it's journaling, breathwork, reframing your thoughts, or talking to a therapist, stick with your practice—even when you don't "feel" it working. Healing often happens silently, beneath the surface, before it becomes visible in your life.

- Accept that some days will be harder than others. Just like the body can feel sore or tired, the mind has days of heaviness. Don't view this as failure. See it as part of the rhythm of healing. Resilience is built through persistence, not perfection.

- Keep showing up for yourself. Even when you slip. Even when you're tired. Showing up again and again sends a message to your brain: "I matter. My wellbeing is worth the effort."

What science says:

Neuroscience confirms that repetition rewires the brain. This process is called neuroplasticity—your brain's ability to change and adapt. The more frequently you practice awareness of your thoughts, emotional regulation, and self-compassion, the stronger those neural pathways become.

Eventually, your mind begins to default to calm instead of chaos, compassion instead of criticism, and hope instead of helplessness.

Healing isn't linear, and it isn't passive. It's a commitment—a decision to return to yourself again and again, even when it's hard. That's what builds mental strength. That's what transforms your story.

Educating your mind: it's not about toxic positivity—it's about inner authority

Educating your mind doesn't mean faking a smile when you're in pain. It's not about ignoring problems or drowning discomfort in cliché affirmations. This isn't toxic positivity—it's conscious mental leadership.

It's about becoming the guardian of your focus, the editor of your internal narrative, and the architect of your emotional responses.

Your mind is a powerful instrument, capable of either spiraling into fear and self-doubt or rising with clarity and resilience. The difference lies in what you choose to feed it.

Every time you choose to respond with calm instead of chaos, truth instead of assumption, or self-compassion instead of self-judgment, you are rewiring your brain. You're carving a new neural pathway—one that tells your mind: "We're safe. We're capable. We're healing."

You don't need to be perfect. You don't need to have it all figured out. But every small act of mental re-education adds up. Every time you pause and reframe a thought, redirect your energy, or breathe through a moment of distress, you're training your mind to support your growth—not sabotage it.

What this means:

- You're not erasing sadness or fear—you're learning how to move through them without being consumed.

- You're not denying reality—you're choosing how to relate to it with wisdom and inner strength.

- You're not broken—you've just been running a mental program that needs updating.

In the next chapter, we'll explore how to protect the progress you've made—so you don't slip back into the same loops of fear, doubt, or emotional burnout. You'll learn how to reinforce the new neural patterns you've begun building and how to create a sustainable mental wellness strategy that adapts with you.

Because the truth is:Your mind isn't broken.It's just been listening to the wrong instructions.Now, you're learning to give it better ones—based on truth, presence, and inner leadership.

Chapter 6

Building emotional resilience

How to sustain a healthy mind for life

You've made it this far, and that alone is proof of your commitment to change. We've explored what depression is, how it impacts your life, and most importantly—how to begin healing. You've learned tools, practices, and mindset shifts that can move you toward clarity, hope, and a sense of control.

But here's the truth: healing isn't just about knowing what to do. It's about learning how to stay well once you've started to feel better.

Many people find relief from depression temporarily, only to spiral again weeks or months later—not because they failed, but because they didn't know how to sustain their progress. And in this chapter, we're going to change that.

You're not here just to survive. You're here to build a life of strength, stability, and resilience.

Why emotional resilience matters

The emotional tools you've gained throughout this journey are like seeds—full of potential, but not yet fully grown. To bloom, they need consistent care, attention, and the right environment. Healing is not a one-time breakthrough; it's a daily decision to show up for yourself with compassion and commitment.

Think of mental health not as a final destination you reach and then forget about, but as an ongoing practice—a way of life. Just like physical fitness, maintaining a healthy mind requires routine effort. Your thoughts, your emotional responses, your habits—they're all trainable. And with practice, they become stronger.

Your mind is your most powerful asset. It's the lens through which you experience every moment of your life. But like any vital part of your being, it needs to be nourished, strengthened, and protected. If left unattended, even the healthiest mind can become vulnerable to fear, self-doubt, and overwhelm.

The good news is: you don't need to be perfect. You don't need to have everything figured out. What you need is willingness—to keep choosing yourself, to return to your tools when things get hard, and to believe that you are capable of building a life that feels good to live.

Yes, you can absolutely create a life where anxiety and depression no longer dominate your days.Yes, you can experience calm within your mind, clarity in your thoughts, and peace in your body.Yes, you can feel connected to your purpose and grounded in your identity.

But this transformation doesn't happen all at once. It unfolds one choice at a time.The choice to rest. The choice to reach out. The choice to speak kindly to yourself.The choice to keep going—especially when you're tempted to give up.

You're not just healing. You're becoming.And now, it's time to learn how to make that healing stick—how to go from knowing what helps to living it every day.

Here's how to sustain your growth and turn mental wellness from a goal into a lifestyle.

1. Make it a daily practice

The tools you've learned—whether journaling, gratitude, therapy, movement, or meditation—aren't one-time fixes. They only work if they become part of your life.

What helps: Create a daily or weekly rhythm that includes at least three positive mental health habits. Don't wait until you "feel like it." Treat them like brushing your teeth—non-negotiable.

2. Trust the process (even when it's slow)

Progress isn't linear. Some days you'll feel light and free. Other days, it may feel like you're back at square one. That's normal. Setbacks don't mean you're broken—they mean you're human.

What helps: Remember that your brain is rewiring. This takes time. Repeat this to yourself: *"I don't have to feel better immediately. I just have to keep showing up."*

3. Practice radical patience

Be gentle with yourself. Depression often comes with high expectations and internal pressure. But healing asks you to slow down, breathe, and allow imperfection.

What helps: When you catch yourself rushing or criticizing your pace, pause and say: *"I am not behind. I'm on my own path."*

4. Curate your circle

You become like the people you surround yourself with. Energy is contagious. Choose wisely.

What helps: Build relationships with people who are kind, open-minded, and growth-oriented. Let go of those who drain you, invalidate your feelings, or encourage old patterns.

5. Stay rooted in your 'why'

Why did you begin this journey? What was your turning point?

Keep that memory close. Write it down. Speak it out loud. Let it be your compass when motivation fades.

What helps: Make a reminder on your phone or a sticky note with your "why"—a phrase that keeps you grounded.

6. Use affirmations as a mental anchor

Affirmations aren't just words—they're cues to remind your brain what's true when the world gets loud.

What helps: Choose 3 affirmations that resonate with your healing. Examples:"I am allowed to take up space.""My past does not define my future.""I am learning to love myself."

Repeat them daily—even if you don't believe them yet. Your brain learns through repetition.

7. Help someone else heal

One of the most empowering ways to deepen your healing is to guide someone else on their journey. When you share what you've learned, you reinforce your own growth.

What helps: Talk to a friend. Post your story online. Volunteer for a mental health cause. Be the light you once needed.

8. Stay open to support

You don't need to do this alone. Sometimes we relapse because we stop reaching out.

What helps: Keep therapy appointments, text a trusted friend, or join a support group. Ask yourself weekly: *"Have I checked in with someone who understands me?"*

9. Make peace a priority, not a perk

Don't wait for peace to "happen." Make it something you actively create.

What helps: Begin each day with a moment of stillness—just one minute of breath, silence, or intention. Train your nervous system to associate calm as your baseline.

10. Accept that setbacks are part of mastery

You may fall. You may forget. But that doesn't mean you've failed.

What helps: Instead of thinking, "I'm back where I started," tell yourself: *"I know how to come back faster now. I'm not starting over—I'm starting stronger."*

You're becoming the phoenix

The most incredible part of healing is not just getting through the dark—it's realizing that you've become someone new because of it. Someone more aware, more conscious, more compassionate.

You don't need to chase perfection. You don't need to control every emotion. You just need to keep choosing to show up for yourself.

So as you continue forward, remember this:

- You are not who you were before.
- You are rising.
- And now—you can rise again and again, no matter what life throws at you.

Depression is a disease—and it must be treated as one. This is not just a matter of willpower or "snapping out of it." It is a real, often chronic condition that affects both the brain and the body, and like any chronic disease, it requires long-term care, understanding, and a thoughtful approach to healing. In my experience working with people facing chronic illnesses, I've seen the same patterns emerge: the journey is rarely straightforward. There are good days and hard days, breakthroughs and setbacks. But through it all, one thing remains constant—there is always work to be done, and there is always hope.

Depression doesn't always have a clear starting point. Sometimes its roots are hidden in the shadows of our early years—moments we don't even consciously remember. Other times, it emerges from more recent pain: a traumatic event, the death of a loved one, an abrupt change, or the slow erosion of our sense of self-worth. Whatever the cause, the symptoms are real. The emptiness, the fatigue, the disconnection, the persistent sadness or numbness—these are not flaws in your character. They are signals.

Depression is the mind and body's way of saying, "Something is out of balance." It is a symptom that your nervous system, your thought patterns, and your emotional core are overwhelmed. The real question is not what is "wrong" with you—but rather, what happened to you, and how can we begin to respond with care and curiosity instead of blame and shame?

Healing begins when you stop fighting yourself and start listening to the signals your body and mind are giving you. Depression is not the end of the story. It is a messenger—a call to reconnect with yourself, to rewrite the patterns that no longer serve you, and to gently return to wholeness.

But this transformation begins with a decision—and only you can make it. You must choose, even on the most difficult days, to show up for yourself. You must be the one to say, "I want to get better. I may not know how, but I'm willing to try." That single act of willingness is powerful. It's not about pretending to be okay—it's about taking responsibility for your healing, step by step, no matter how small.

No one else can do this work for you. Others can walk beside you, support you, guide you—but the decision to change, to seek healing, to choose life over despair—it has to start inside of you.

You are not broken. You are responding to pain in the only way your system knew how at the time. But now, you have new tools. You have awareness. You have support. And you have the ability to begin again—every single day.

Because you are not your depression. You are the one strong enough to face it—and heal.

Conclusion

Becoming the healer of your own mind

Thank you for walking this journey with me. The fact that you've made it to the end of this book already says so much about your strength, courage, and determination. I want you to pause and acknowledge that—you didn't give up. You kept reading. You stayed open. And that's no small thing.

Isn't it incredible that something you've been silently battling for weeks, months, or even years—depression—can begin to loosen its grip through the most grounded, human methods? Breathing. Feeling. Observing. Choosing again. So often, we overcomplicate life when, in truth, healing thrives in simplicity.

Depression and anxiety are not life sentences. They are signals—calls from your inner self begging to be heard, honored, and understood. And once you've recognized them for what they are, you take your power back.

Throughout this book, I've invited you to challenge the beliefs that have kept you stuck, to observe your internal dialogue with compassion, and to rewire your thought patterns one step at a time. Everything shared with you here was born from years of work with real people—patients, survivors, humans just like you—who faced unimaginable pain: abuse, betrayal, loss, trauma. Some carried wounds so deep, I wondered if the light would ever return to their eyes. And yet, many of them did heal. Not overnight. Not without effort. But over time—with courage, tools, and the unshakable decision to heal—they rose.

The one thing they all had in common? They stopped waiting to feel ready. They stopped waiting for the pain to disappear. They simply decided to begin. That decision changed everything.

So now the question is: what will you do with all you've learned?

It's not enough to read this book and place it back on the shelf. Knowledge is only the beginning. True healing comes when you apply it. Many people keep searching for answers—books, podcasts, seminars—yet they remain trapped, not because they don't know what to do, but because they don't **do** what they know.

You cannot heal if you treat this wisdom like optional advice. You must embody it. Integrate it. Breathe life into it through consistent action.

If you need to monitor your thoughts daily, do it. If certain environments, people, or habits pull you back into darkness—cut them off. No apology is needed when protecting your peace. Prioritize your mental health the way you would your oxygen. Without it, nothing else works.

You are no longer the person who feels powerless. You have the tools now. It's time to use them.

Write a plan. Schedule healing into your day like a sacred ritual. Talk to someone. Move your body. Nourish your mind. Protect your energy. Most importantly, make a vow to yourself—that no matter how heavy the days feel, you will keep going. Not perfectly. Not without struggle. But with intention.

And when fear whispers that you're not strong enough, speak louder:"I am healing. I am worthy. I am not alone."

You do not have to fight every thought. You do not have to win every battle today. You simply have to keep showing up for yourself.

The world becomes a better place when people heal. You will become a better parent, partner, friend, professional—not by hiding your wounds, but by tending to them. Your healing ripples outward.

I cannot wait to hear your story. I look forward to the day when you, too, are guiding someone else through the dark—because you made it through.

Until then, I leave you with this:

You are *brave enough to begin again.* You are *strong enough to rise.* You are *already becoming who you were always meant to be.*

And remember:

You are brave. You are happy. You are strong. You are home.

A note about Hypnocell®

As you continue your healing journey, I want to share a powerful resource that may support you further.

I created Hypnocell® as an integrative method to restore the connection between mind and body—a connection that often becomes disrupted in states of chronic stress, trauma, and depression. This method blends hypnosis, neuroscience, and cellular regeneration tools to help individuals access the deeper root of emotional distress and begin the process of rewiring both the subconscious mind and nervous system.

Depression is not just a chemical imbalance—it's often the result of unresolved emotional trauma, limiting beliefs, and the body being stuck in survival mode. Hypnocell® offers techniques that go beyond surface-level treatment and help your system return to a state of safety, clarity, and repair.

Through guided sessions, mind-body education, and personalized support, Hypnocell® has helped many people shift from merely surviving to thriving. It's not a replacement for therapy or medical care—but a complementary, holistic tool that supports your nervous system in doing what it was designed to do: heal.

If you feel drawn to explore this further, I invite you to visit www.hypnocell.com to learn more.

You don't have to do it all alone. Tools exist. Help exists. And you are worth every step toward wholeness.

About the author

Dr. Lucy Coleman is a medical doctor, neuroscientist, and integrative mind-body practitioner who has spent over 15 years helping individuals navigate the complex path of healing—physically, emotionally, and mentally.

Trained in reproductive medicine and hypnosis, and the creator of the Hypnocell® Method, Dr. Coleman blends science with the subtle intelligence of the subconscious mind. Her work is grounded in one fundamental truth: that the human body and mind are deeply connected—and that true healing begins when we treat them as such.

But this book isn't written only from clinical knowledge. It's also born from personal experience.

There was a time in her life when depression took hold—quietly at first, like an invisible fog, until it clouded her confidence, energy, and sense of purpose. Like many, she tried to carry on as if nothing was wrong. But the weight became too much.

What changed everything was learning to listen to her body. To decode the messages behind the symptoms. To understand that depression wasn't a weakness—but a signal. It asked for her attention, her compassion, and her willingness to change the way she related to herself.

Even today, she admits that there are still moments when the shadows return. But now, she no longer fears them. With the tools she teaches in this book—and in her Hypnocell® program—she knows how to meet those moments with strength, awareness, and calm.

Her mission is to share what she's learned so that others don't have to suffer in silence or confusion. Through writing, speaking, and guiding others one-on-one, Dr. Coleman helps people reconnect to their inner resilience and build lives rooted in clarity, peace, and purpose.

You can learn more about her method and resources at www.hypnocell.com.

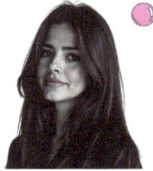

Thank you for taking the time to read this book. Whether you're just starting your journey or have already taken steps toward healing, please know: I see your courage, your strength, and your willingness to grow. That alone is a powerful sign that change is possible—and already underway.

If this book has helped you shift your perspective, feel more supported, or take even one small step toward balance, I would love to hear from you.

Share your experience and leave a review—your words could inspire someone else to take the first step too.

You can also reach out to me directly to let me know how you're doing or where you are in your journey. Your story matters.

Continue your journey with us

For deeper support, tools, and healing practices, I invite you to explore:

LifeBossHealth

My mind-body health platform offering science-based programs and emotional wellness tools to help you reclaim your vitality and personal power.

Hypnocell®

A neuroscience-based method I developed that uses hypnosis, guided visualization, and subconscious reprogramming to promote deep healing, emotional regulation, and mind-body alignment.It has helped countless patients find relief from chronic emotional pain—and it may help you too.

Let's stay connected

Follow me on Instagram for more inspiration, videos, and wellness tools.You'll also find updates about new resources, live sessions, and community spaces where you can feel supported and heard.

You don't have to walk this path alone.Thank you again for allowing me to be part of your journey.

With all my support,

Dr. Lucy Coleman

www.ingramcontent.com/pod-product-compliance
Lightning Source LLC
Chambersburg PA
CBHW041225270326
41934CB00001B/7